HYPNOSIS, HEADACHE AND PAIN CONTROL

An Indirect Approach

by

Stuart W. Bassman, Ed.D.
William C. Wester, II, Ed.D.

Copyright © 1984
Ohio Psychology Publishing Co.
5 E. Long St., Suite 610
Columbus, Ohio 43215

Adapted from: Hypnosis and pain control, in *Clinical hypnosis: A multidisciplinary approach,* W. C. Wester, II, Ed.D., and A. H. Smith, Jr. (eds.), Philadelphia, Lippincott, 1984.

Library of Congress Cataloging in Publication Data

Bassman, Stuart W., 1949–
   Hypnosis, headache, and pain control.

   Bibliography: p.
   Includes index.
   1. Headache—Treatment. 2. Hypnotism—Therapeutic use.
3. Pain—Treatment. I. Wester, William C. II. Title.
RB128.B37   1984   616.8'49   84-2172
ISBN 0-910707-05-7

*Dedicated
to
Joan
and
Betty*

Table of Contents

INTRODUCTION

In the last 40 years the treatment of pain has gone through a number of up-heavals. World War II brought a pharmacological revolution in alleviating and reducing pain. With an avalanche of injuries and casualties and a shortage of doctors and nurses, drugs appeared to be the buffer between agonizing suffering and time for a cure. Yet, drug use became drug abuse, as addiction, side effects, and in some cases the cure, became the curse.

In the last decade, efforts to find non-drug alternatives of treatment have in-creased. The short term goal has not only been to cure, but also to help alleviate a sufferer's pain without detriment to that person's physical and psychological health. The treatments presented in this book are safe procedures, shown to be successful in effecting relief from several painful maladies (Bassman, 1983).

These procedures were designed to provide a safe and effective method of relief for individuals suffering from one type of chronic pain condition — muscle-con-traction headache. According to Beatty and Haynes (1979), 20 to 30% of the general population suffer from this malady. The experimental and clinical applica-tions of this therapy involved adult women who had experienced muscle-contrac-tion or tension headaches for a 2-year period. The success of a comprehensive experimental study utilizing these treatments by Bassman (1983) insures that they may be considered a viable alternative to drugs and surgery for the relief of pain. In the words of Hippocrates, ". . . nothing should be omitted in an art which interests the whole world, one which may be beneficial to suffering humanity and which does not risk human life or comfort" (Kroger, 1979). Thus, the goal of these treatments is to alleviate pain and suffering associated with muscle-contraction headache.

In general, the treatments consist of the use of "indirect" hypnosis, meaning subtle suggestion, to help subjects relax and increase their responsiveness to an idea or set of ideas (suggestions), to reduce their headache activity. These pro-cedures are operationally defined by four scripts standardizing the treatments. Each of the actual scripts begins with a different induction, used as a cue to relax, and containing suggestions related to the therapeutic goal. Also included in these procedures are instructions for developing imagery, along with using metaphors and analogies to deepen the hypnotic trance. Further, suggestions are offered for headache reduction, ego strenghtening, coping strategies and glove anesthesia. The control of headache activity by the patient is achieved in a gradual fashion, with a greater percentage of pain being brought under control during each succes-sive session. The scripts are created by drawing on the works of Bandler and Grinder, 1975, 1977; Bressler, 1979; Erickson, 1959, 1968; Haley, 1967, 1973; Hartland, 1966, 1971; and Zeig, 1980. Use was also made of the model scripts presented in *A syllabus on hypnosis and a handbook of therapeutic suggestions* (The American Society of Clinical Hypnosis, Education and Research, 1973).

FIRST SESSION

FIRST SESSION

COMMENT

INDUCTION

Therapist establishing:

— *Rapport*

— *Interest*

— *Empathy*

— *Positive response set*

"Before we begin, I am going to outline to you what will happen during this session and how well you will do. You may view this as seeing a preview before investing in a movie. This preview will include my getting to know more about you. I'll ask you some questions that will help me so that I may help you.

"Next, we will discuss your present problem and how you have dealt with it. Then, we will discuss your ideas and concepts of hypnosis, and then discuss what hypnosis is, and how *your* use of it will help you. A little later, whenever you are ready to enter a pleasant and deep hypnotic state, you can let me know — after all, you will be the one in control. And you will learn that all hypnosis is actually self-hypnosis, but we will come back to that later."

COMMENT

The therapist then helps patients to feel more at ease, as they are encouraged to discuss those aspects of their lives they feel most comfortable sharing. Subsequently, the therapist will gradually focus on patients' maladies and how they have dealt with them. It is essential that the therapist be empathetic regarding patients' reactions to their pain. This is especially crucial with headache sufferers, as these people are quite sensitive to others' reactions to their ailment. People with chronic headaches are often defensive about their pain, while those close to them react with disbelief or irritation. The professional should be acutely sensitive to this issue. One way of understanding the situation is to note that whatever is painful for an individual is the ultimate criterion of the value ascribed to it. So for patients, the pain is real if they believe it is. In addition, through initially reinforcing patients' belief in their perception of pain, the professional also provides a framework (hypnosis) for changing their experience of pain.

The session proceeds as the therapist discusses with patients their concepts and possible misconceptions about hypnosis. Most individuals perceive hypnosis as having a mystique which they feel ambivalent about. It is essential for the professional to discuss and assure patients about what hypnosis is and is not. This also provides the therapist with the added opportunity to align patients' expectations with their conception of how self-hypnosis will help them.

The reader may note that a consistent pattern develops, wherein the professional emphasizes and models to patients an attitude of empathy, patient responsibility and control of their perceptions, and how their utilization of hypnosis will help them when they are ready to be helped.

COMMENT

Emphasis on patient control, and relaxing, non-threatening atmosphere. The manner and the mood of the therapist should convey a feeling of re-assurance that patients will do very well.

INDUCTION

"That's right, get as comfortable in the chair as you would like. While you are getting settled and relaxed, I'm going to show you how you will go into a very pleasant trance, O.K.? . . . yes. I want you to enjoy being very comfortable. Let me do the work, you can just relax.

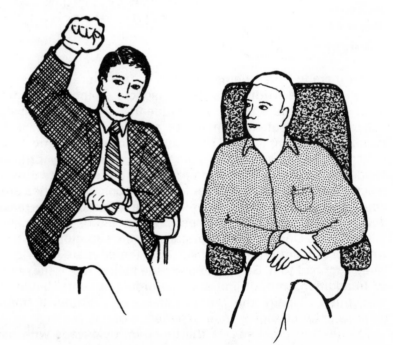

Therapist models concentration on one focal point.

COMMENT	INDUCTION
Therapist models behavior of being a good subject, and also prepares patients for what to expect; may lessen their anxiety by knowing what to do and how easy it will be. *A rationale is offered defining this as a collaborative approach.*	"Now, just watch me. In a little while, when you are ready to begin at your own pace and your own rate, just raise one of your arms. Whichever arm you prefer to use. You are the one in control, and so the choice will be up to you. Now I'm raising my right arm just above my eye level. I am then clenching my fist, and as you notice, I'm staring at my fist. "Now let me explain the rationale and importance of what I am doing. There are four reasons associated with our approach. First, it demonstrates your ability to concentrate your energy and tension into one focal point, your hand. Second, the natural consequence of focusing your energy into part of your body will cause that part to tense, begin to strain, and become uncomfortable — even painful. However, we frequently overlook what is very obvious — our natural ability to correct this unpleasantness by *allowing* ourselves to blink our eyes and then to close them as they tire from the strain of staring at our fist. As we do, correspondingly our tight fist begins to loosen effortlessly, and the focused tension begins to decrease as our hand lowers gently to our lap. Of course, this is very natural and comfortable.
Therapist should note if patients blink eyes when he/she says this. This is an indication of how open they are to this experience.	
Therapist's hand begins to descend. Softer voice. *Therapist is modeling how to be very relaxed and at ease.*	"The third reason we do this is because you will learn to associate these natural occurrences with going into a very deep, helpful, and pleasant trance state. For you, your hand will symbolize a lever that you can use to control the depth of your comfortable trance. So as your hand — or lever — goes down, your eyes will blink, then close, and then *you* will control your descent into a very relaxing and pleasant hypnotic state. All I will be doing is talking — and all you need to do is to relax — very, very deeply. That sounds O.K., doesn't it? Yes.

COMMENT	INDUCTION

COMMENT

Therapist gazes thought-fully, thus encouraging patient imagination and also emphasizing patient sovereignty over self.

Being calm and unhurried can be reassuring to patients. If patients indicate they are ready to begin and yet therapist continues to diligently prepare them, it may increase their willingness to experience a trance state.

Focusing on the immediate experience that we usually ignore can add to therapist's credibility and also can be used as a means of developing a trance.

At this point, some patients may still be apprehensive about starting by exhibiting some stalling tactics (numerous questions, etc.).

INDUCTION

"The fourth reason for using this approach is so you will learn how to control a focal point of tension or energy, and transform it into relaxation — or perhaps just a comforting, gentle experience.

"I don't know what the limits are, of what you can make it, mmmm. . . . It is entirely up to *you,* just by utilizing self-hypnosis.

"So you will be in control. And by using self-hypnosis, you *will* be able to control a portion of, or all of you, if that is what *you decide!*

"Any questions before you will go into a trance? (Be reassuring, if patients have any questions. Always use a positive response set in answering patients. For example: "It's good that you feel skeptical about going into a trance. It is a sign of intelligence to doubt, and will only make you a better subject"; or "By your affirming that you are ready to begin and don't have any questions, you indicate that you are highly motivated and will really benefit from self-hypnosis, and will be an excellent participant. Good!")

"Now, if anyone comes to the door, or if the phone rings, just leave it to me. I know you can hear any sounds that you wish (slowly mention sounds in immediate environment), but actually the only important thing right now is the sound of my voice and the meaning of what I have to say to you, so you really don't need to give any attention to anything else unless you have a particular interest in . . . (refer to sounds already mentioned).

"So now whenever you are ready to enter a pleasant hypnotic state, simply raise your arm, clench your fist tightly, and mobilize that tension through your entire body right into your hand." Wait until patient begins to

Therapist should respond by continuing to be permissive and empathetic by perhaps discussing patients' expectations and feelings.

move hand and then say: "That's right! Feel that tension move from the tip of your head and from the bottom of your toes. All that tension, energy, coming to a head in your shoulder, your arm, your hand!" Gently elevate the patient's fist above eye level, making sure that it is rigid. While doing this, say:

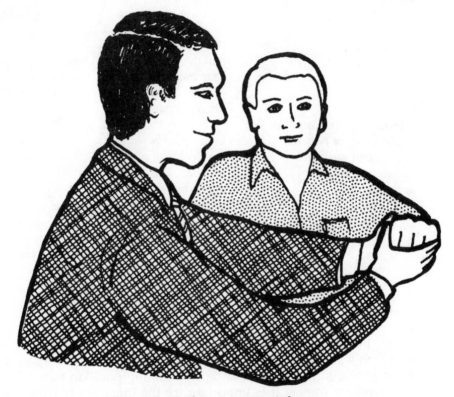

Therapist induces arm catalepsy.

Therapist induces arm catalepsy.

"Here, let me show you. Your shoulder, your arm, your hand are becoming very hard, like a steel beam or iron girder is running through them. So hard! Good! Get in touch with that rigidity, steel. That's right, begin to stare at it, so you can watch what is happening, as you experience yourself going into a deep hyp-

-5-

Predicting what will happen when patients are ready to allow it provides increased credibility for therapist.

Therapist gives plausible explanation of patients' self-control over their autonomic nervous systems.

notic trance. Because your hand will tire of the struggle and loosen its grip, you will feel this weariness spread throughout all of you. What was once tension, straining and discomfort will become comfortable and pleasant, and you will experience yourself *melting* into the chair — perhaps like butter, *melting* into the chair. Now, I don't know how much tension is in your body, or how long it will take to centralize in your hand, but there is plenty of time, plenty of time — like butter, melting into the chair — softly, at your own pace and your own rate. After all, you are the one in control. Plenty of time, plenty of time . . . (therapist pauses).

"Even as you are sitting in that chair, you have probably not realized it yet, but already the rhythm of your breathing has changed. It is slower, it is more comfortable, and it is a good rhythm! Your whole bodily process is changing to meet your new level of comfort. Your blood pressure is lowering, your heartbeat is at a comfortable range. I want you to enjoy being very comfortable — whenever you are ready, whenever you are ready."

COMMENT

The therapist should not be preoccupied with patients' progress at this point. After all, this situation has been structured so that when patients lower their hands to a resting position they will be in a hypnotic trance. It is important for the therapist to insure arm catalepsy, so that patients will necessarily have to lower their arms, whether after a very brief or longer period of time. It can also be reaffirming to patients that the therapist is indeed keeping his/her word to "allow" patients control over themselves. The therapist is thereby reinforcing, by this behavior, a belief in the sovereignty of the patients over themselves. A patient might be concerned about the issue of responsibility and control of oneself. Some patients may believe that if the pain is out of their control, they are thus not responsible for the pain and its effects on their lives.

One of the essential elements of this treatment, however, is that people regain responsibility for themselves and have the opportunity of regulating their perception of pain. So, rather than debating the authenticity of the pain, the therapist affirms perception of the pain, but also emphasizes that it is *their* perception, which can be changed by utilizing self-hypnosis.

COMMENT

Therapist gives familiar examples to patients to help them feel at ease; communicates to patients in a reassuring manner.

INDUCTION

"In a sense, what we are doing here corresponds to what happens when you have a doctor listen to the sound of your heart beating. The doctor does not discover your heartbeat, but by the use of a stethoscope is able to become aware of your heartbeat. That is what we will be doing with hypnosis, becoming aware of the vast potential of something quite natural that is always going on inside of you — something you are capable of doing, that you are vaguely aware of. Now, you will be able to control your ability to experience and utilize the benefits of the relaxing and deeply pleasant feelings that are deep . . . deep . . . inside of you. These feelings are always with you, it's just that sometimes we ignore the obvious." (At this point, refer to whatever behavior patient is exhibiting, and note how this indicates entering into a deep hypnotic state; i.e., "Good, you are swallowing, staring, smiling, etc. That indicates you are getting more and more deeply, deeply relaxed."

COMMENT

It is important for the therapist to be reassuring and not get involved in a struggle if patients have difficulty entering the trance state. The therapist should keep using patients' behavior as a starting point for demonstrating that they are doing very well. *Be with the patient!* Some other ways of doing this are:

"As you smile (or other behavior), you feel yourself becoming more and more relaxed (pause). As you listen to the sound of my voice, you feel yourself becoming more and more relaxed (pause). It is fine to smile (or other behavior). Smiling (other behavior) is a way of relaxing, and it is a pleasant experience. Yes. After all, you are the one in control. Plenty of time, plenty of time (pause). You are doing very well. Good."

COMMENT

It is also very helpful to synchronize your hypnotic words with clients' exhalations of breath. Watch patients' shoulders, which will lower when they exhale, and follow their rhythm. When patients exhale, you exhale in a breathy voice with such words as: relax, deep, deeper, restful, comfortable, peaceful.

COMMENT

Age regression to very early learning experience, where children are initially taught different ways of expressing themselves.

Therapist continues to emphasize that whatever patients are feeling are their own unique ways of experiencing hypnosis.

Countdown is introduced both as a cognitive mode of deepening a trance and as an additional method of relaxation, to the physical

INDUCTION

"It's interesting — when I see (or saw, if hand is already down) your hand up, it reminds me of when I was a child in school. I remember my teacher explaining to our class that in order to be recognized and acknowledged, one needs to raise an arm, and wait until the teacher calls his name. Well, I was a little confused about this procedure, but it seemed to be the right thing to do. After all, I was there to learn, and this was my first lesson. That's right (patient's name), relax very, very deeply.

"Well, the teacher would say my name and I would lower my hand. Kind of silly, but it worked, (patient's name). Good. Just keep on allowing yourself to melt into the chair. Just let yourself be very comfortable and peaceful. I'll simply keep on talking and you can become so deeply relaxed (pause), so calm (pause), so comfortable (pause). No need for you to speak now, just enjoy the really comforting feelings you are experiencing.

"Just to help you relax even more deeply, in a little while I am going to count down from ten to one. As you hear the numbers going down, feel yourself going deeper and deeper. I know some people imagine themselves going

-8-

COMMENT	INDUCTION

one previously used.

down an elevator, or escalator, or a flight of stairs. I don't know what you will imagine as I count down from ten to one, but you will feel yourself becoming more and more peaceful, calm and comfortable. As the numbers go down, you feel your relaxation going up. Good.

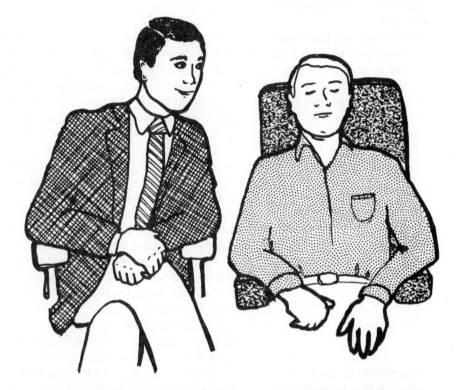

Therapist observes the rhythm of patient's breathing.

The therapist should watch the rhythm of patients' breathing by observing their shoulders rising with inhalation and lowering with exhalation. Therapist says each number as patients exhale, in his/her

"Ten . . . nine, deeper and deeper, at your own rate and at your own pace . . . eight, restful, in control . . . seven, more and more deeply relaxed . . . six, calm, a full person in every way . . . five, halfway there, you are doing very well, good . . . four (soft voice) . . . three, gently, peacefully, comfortable . . . twoooo, deeper and deeper, and one, good!

COMMENT

own breathy voice, again reinforcing patients' being comfortable in experiencing their own inner world. Then, the therapist adds that patients are free to exert inner control by simply changing their posture (perceptions).

From this point, the therapist may help patients to a deeper level of relaxation by simply slurring the "s" at the end of certain words. For instance, "yes" becomes "yesss."

Very vague, general statements so that patients can define an experience for their own benefit.

INDUCTION

Now, as you are sitting there in a relaxed state, feeling very much at ease and at peace with yourself, I want you to enjoy feeling very comfortable. For example, if at any time you need to readjust your posture to help yourself feel more deeply relaxed and more at ease, do so; after all, you are the one in control.

"In fact, perhaps you can allow yourself to become aware of how relaxed and comfortable you are. Of course, you can allow your conscious mind to relax, and comfortably and pleasantly think about a very calm and restful place, your favorite peaceful place. It's entirely up to you. Do this at your own rate and at your own pace. Good. And you can enjoy this so much that you can let your unconscious mind listen to me while your conscious mind can continue to deeply relax. Deeply — for after all your unconscious mind will remember what is important for you to know. That's right; you are doing very well, yesss.

"Now, many of the things I want to assist you in accomplishing are governed by your unconscious mind. Continue as you are, at ease, in comfort, relaxing very peacefully, and at the right time you will become aware of how to take care of your concerns, all of those that you need to deal with here.

"Now, I am going to discuss your problem and I believe you will be comfortable with the way I present it to you. I will sketch it in general and I want you to realize that I am going to ask of you only the things that are actually possible for you to do. There are many things that we can do about which we are unaware. As I told you before, I will ask you to do only those things that you are capable of doing. The question is, how much are you really capable of controlling in your body?

COMMENT	INDUCTION

COMMENT

Therapist is defining the functioning of the autonomic nervous system, and then introducing the concept of the unconscious.

Age regression using familiar examples for most people.

Therapist should always use him- or herself as a model to encourage age regression.

While patients are relaxing, the therapist presents a pleasant analogy which essentially outlines the therapeutic style that will be used in this endeavor.

INDUCTION

"Now, if I were to ask you how each of your internal organs, such as your heart, your lungs, or even perhaps how your head functions, you might find it difficult to explain. But now, as I speak to you, all of the parts of your body are functioning quite well without your understanding exactly how they operate. So it is not really necessary for you to know how your body works; it is on automatic pilot, but there must always be a pilot.

"In your lifetime of experience, you have felt some things and you have not felt other things because you chose not to. You have had much experience in forgetting things that would seem upon ordinary thinking to be unforgettable.

"I remember being in school on some (describe present weather outside) days. I would frequently daydream when I got tired of the teacher's lecturing. I used to like sitting by the window, so I could always look outside, and wonder — Mmm. There would always be something pleasant to dream about, no matter what was going on in the room. And maybe I was looking forward to a birthday party, or going somewhere, going to visit Grandma, or going on a trip.

"I don't know what you're thinking, but I remember (pause) playing in the yard (pause), in the school yard (pause), looking forward to vacation time, and really having a good time.

"I remember my teacher telling us stories all the time; I would enjoy that, and even remember some of them. Once there was a disagreement between the North Wind and the Sun. The North Wind boasted of being the more powerful; the Sun merely smiled. Just then a traveler came into sight, and they agreed to test the matter by trying to see which of them could make the traveler remove his coat. The pompous North Wind was the first to try, while the Sun watched from

COMMENT	INDUCTION

behind a gray cloud. The North Wind blew a furious blast and nearly tore the coat from its fastenings; but the traveler only held the coat closer in desperation. The North Wind was surprised by this resistance and its fearsome gales were soon spent. Shocked by the traveler's resiliency, the Wind withdrew in despair. 'I don't believe you can do it either, mighty Sun.' Then out came the kindly Sun in all its splendor, dispelling the clouds that had gathered and sending warm and refreshing

Therapist slowly enunciates each part of the body.

rays down upon the traveler's head (pause), neck (pause), shoulders (pause), chest (pause), stomach (pause), legs (pause), and feet. The traveler smiled at experiencing such a wondrous spring day, and thought that this was surely a day to take off a coat and to greet the spring (pause). That's fine, you're relaxing very deeply.

Development of new association, one of calmness, relaxation. Reinforcement that change will occur, and it is up to patients to become aware of it.

"Now, you have the wonderful opportunity to associate relaxation of your body and mind with a very comfortable attitude. For already the pattern of your headaches is changing. I'm not sure if the change will be gradual or occur rather quickly. You see, we frequently overlook the gradual changes and are all too aware of the swift ones. Yes, sometimes we even overlook the minute changes unless someone brings them to our attention. Hmmm — it is occurring even now as you sit comfortably in the chair. For after all, that's the reason you are here, so that your headaches will become less severe, less frequent and, of course, won't last as long. And they will leave, when you decide they will!

Emphasis on patient responsibility.

"That's right, relax very deeply. Good, you're doing well. I want you to enjoy being very comfortable.

Once again, patients are challenged to become aware of forthcoming changes and effects.

"I don't know what changes you will become aware of first, maybe in the severity of the pain, perhaps in the duration of time, I don't know, maybe in frequency. You might

COMMENT	INDUCTION

INDUCTION

not even be aware of the changes while they are occurring, but you will be aware of the effects. Yes, that's right.

"For after all, you are much more than a headache, much more (pause). Relax very deeply. There's so much for you to become aware of, so much for you to become aware of. I want you to enjoy being very comfortable. From now on, you have the wonderful opportunity to associate relaxation of your body and mind with a very comfortable attitude.

Therapist clearly enunciates number "ten." Sometimes patients come out of the trance without having their hands rise; this in no way indicates

"In a few moments, I will count from one to ten. When I say the number ten your hand will begin to rise, the same hand you used as a lever to place yourself in a trance. However, this time your hand will rise up, at your own pace and at your own rate, and when it

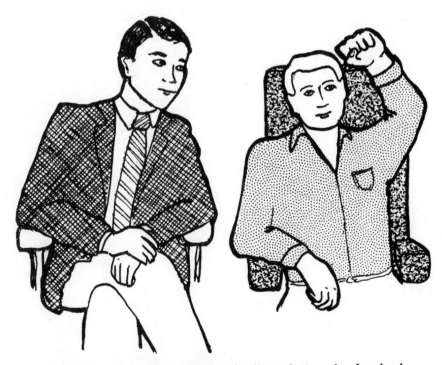

Patient comes out of trance feeling alert and refreshed.

COMMENT	INDUCTION

COMMENT

that they were not in a trance.

INDUCTION

reaches the same level from where it started when you first raised your hand, you will open your eyes and come out of the trance feeling alert, refreshed and also very relaxed as if you had just experienced a very peaceful, soothing and comforting nap.

"Tonight, when you go to sleep, you will be able to really enjoy the comfort of your bed. You will have a deep and restful sleep, like one you had a long, long time ago. And you will awaken in the morning feeling calm, secure, rested, comfortable, and confident. Yes, you will be confident of your ability to easily go into and come out of a trance, and to comfortably carry out this treatment and to reap the benefits. Good. Easier and easier. You are doing very well.

Therapist starts counting slowly and softly, then at "five" increases volume and tempo.

"Now, one (pause), two (pause), three (pause), four (pause), five (pause), six, seven, eight, nine, and *ten*. Now it is up to you, at your own pace and at your own rate. Good."

SECOND SESSION

SECOND SESSION

COMMENT

In this session, as in those to follow, patients should be informed about any forthcoming changes in procedures. It is important that patients experience this relationship as collaborative. The rationale for this is to emphasize the patients' being active and responsible partners. The effects of the treatments will need to be maintained after the actual treatment sessions end, which will be accomplished by continued patient activity.

The therapist should inform patients that today they will first discuss anything significant either directly or indirectly related to the treatment which has transpired since they were last together. This may include any changes in headaches, greater ability to relax after the last session, a deeper sleep than usual, or anything else that may be relevant. The therapist should record any changes reported by patients, and then emphasize to patients that changes are already happening. Even changes in depth of relaxation during the last session, or being motivated enough to stay in the treatment should be reinforced. This becomes evidence of the posthypnotic suggestion at the end of the first treatment session, that patients will experience some changes, perhaps small at first, that will increase and eventually add up.

Review of reactions to treatment since last session: "How are you today?" "Have there been any changes in headaches, sleep patterns, daily activities?", etc.

Therapist should note patients' reactions to last induction, remembering to reinforce any positive reactions and to avoid what patients dislike. If applicable, therapist should ask if patients 1) have practiced at all, 2) have recorded practices, and 3) are still self-monitoring.

In preparation for second session, therapist should inform patients that this will be a different induction, with more options to choose from. Therapist should describe induction procedure.

After proceding through the initial phase, as described above, it is time for the second session to begin.

COMMENT   **INDUCTION**

Pre induction.   "That's right, get as comfortable in the chair as you would like. I'm going to demon-

COMMENT	INDUCTION

strate another induction technique you can use to develop a very deep and pleasant hypnotic trance. Just watch me. That's all,

Reassuring.

you will be able to do this very well. Yes. In a little while, whenever you are ready to enter a trance, all you will need to do will be to clasp your hands together tightly in front of you.

Therapist demonstrates.

Once you have them clasped together, begin to exert tension in that area. That's right, just like you did when you raised your arm the last time. However, this time you will feel the force straining from both of your arms. As you can see, my hands are tightly pressed against each other. I am also watching them closely. In a

Patients may be staring at therapist's hands and already experiencing some degree of relaxation.

little while, my hands, my arms, my shoulders, my eyes will tire from the strain and want to relax. Now, I don't know how long this will take. It really doesn't matter how long. But it will happen. First, my fingers will stop straining and tensing and they will begin to loosen, then my hands will loosen. It will be a little difficult for my fingers and hands to come apart. They will feel as if they were stuck together, but they will begin to come apart. That's right. As they do, I will correspondingly feel my eyes blinking and eventually closing, and then my hands will come to rest in my lap. It is very relaxing. This very

Therapist uses very soft voice.

pleasant feeling will travel throughout your body, as if your bloodstream had a soothing, refreshing, calming effect. Of course, I will be talking the whole time you are doing this, and at times you may feel as if my speech pattern matches the rhythm of your relaxation. That's fine. I will then count down from ten to one,

Once again, therapist informs and reassures patients of what to expect.

just to help you go even deeper and become more relaxed, and then I will continue talking until it's time for you to come out of the trance feeling very, very good.

"Any questions before you go into a trance?"

COMMENT

Once again, it is important to encourage a positive response set for patients. Use a tone, mood and attitude that conveys a supportive, reassuring message that patients will succeed. Keep on "being with the patients." Remember to use patients' behavior, attitudes, feelings, even skepticism as either a starting point or the effect of being good subjects. Also, any feedback from patients as to what they liked and disliked in the previous induction; i.e., words, scenes, voice quality, etc. will be useful additions to this induction. Being aware of the present emotional state of patients may also be helpful. Modifying your style to reflect patients' unique characteristics can only add more credibility to your induction.

COMMENT

Patients are becoming sensitized to therapist's use of environment, and by just focusing their attention are becoming more relaxed.

Therapist stares at hands.

Therapist communicates a feeling of reassurance and excitement.

Patient responsibility for developing self-tension and

INDUCTION

"Now, if anyone comes to the door, or if the phone rings, just leave it to me. I know that you can hear any sounds that you wish (slowly mention sounds presently in environment); but, actually the only important thing for you right now is the sound of my voice and the meaning of what I have to say to you, so you really don't need to give any attention to anything else unless you have a particular interest in (refer to sounds already mentioned).

"So whenever you are ready to enter a pleasant hypnotic state, simply clasp your hands tightly. Mobilize that tension throughout your body right into your hands. (Wait till patients begin to move their hands and then say) That's right! Feel that tension, energy, force flow from all of you and come to a head in these hands. Focus your attention on what is happening — that's right — watch what happens. I know some people imagine that each of their hands symbolizes an opposing force. Perhaps one hand represents a wish for something and the other hand represents a power denying the wish. It is up to you what you think about, as your hands press hard against each other. After all, you are the one in control!

"One of the reasons we use this approach for going into a hypnotic trance is that you

COMMENT	INDUCTION

COMMENT

self-hypnosis.

INDUCTION

can watch yourself create a strain, a tension, and then be able to transform it into a very pleasant relaxed state. It really isn't necessary for you to speak, just experience whatever is going on inside you. I will be right here with you. So experience whatever you need to in order to relax . . . deeply. I don't know how much tension is in your body or how long it will take you to centralize it in your hands, but we have plenty of time.

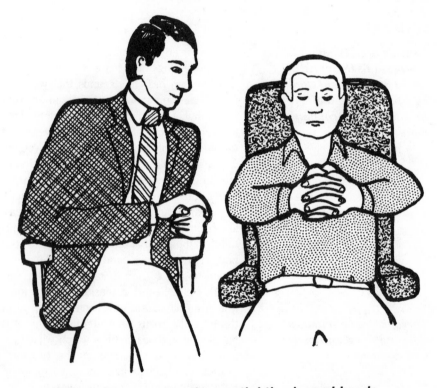

Patient focuses attention on tightly clasped hands.

Therapist creates curiosity, anticipation for what will happen.

"Now, whenever you are ready to go deeply into a hypnotic trance and let go of the tension, simply allow your fingers to come apart, your hands to let go — and eventually settle comfortably in your lap — and then your eyes

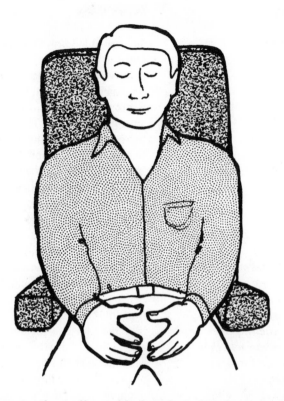

As he relaxes, patient allows his hands to let go and rest in his lap.

will close and you will be in a comfortable relaxed state.

"You will feel very relaxed and experience a deep and pleasant trance state.

"You will come out feeling really good, relaxed, and confident in your ability to do this without me. After all, all hypnosis is self-hypnosis. I am merely showing you how you will help yourself.

"Perhaps at first you might find it a little difficult to separate your fingers from each other. When you are ready to go deeper, they may feel stuck together, but that's O.K., all you will need to do is merely let go.

Therapist graciously leads into a story that essentially focuses on an internal

"I was talking to someone the other day about letting go, and he told me an interesting story. It seems that there is a certain kind of

COMMENT	INDUCTION

COMMENT

struggle.

*Therapist's delivery
should be slow with
emphasis on pacing
patients' breathing.
It is up to the thera-
pist's discretion whether
to enliven the imagery
for patients.*

*Moral of the story em-
phasizes the importance
of being aware of an
internal conflict.*

*Therapist uses whichever
is appropriate.*

INDUCTION

monkey found only in China. These rare and valuable animals are called "rice monkeys," because they love rice. For a long time, no one knew how to catch these lovely animals. A group of animal lovers, however, devised an ingenious plan. They cut small holes in the center of several coconuts, large enough to hold a small amount of rice and a monkey's hand. Then, they decided they would leave a number of these enticing coconuts lying on the jungle floor and then wait, hidden from view. The rice monkeys would then come down from their trees, attracted by the aroma of the rice. They knew that they were quicker than anyone, so even if someone came, the monkeys could still scurry away.

"Now, the monkeys easily fit their hands into the coconuts to get the rice, but once they had the rice in their grip, their hands were larger than the holes, and thus they were not able to take them out. You can imagine the squealing monkeys, gyrating and jumping up and down, struggling to get these coconuts off! Now, the animal lovers just had to come along, merely lift up the coconuts and attached to each one was a yelping monkey — mmmm, some scene!

"If only the monkeys had realized that all they needed to do was to let go of the rice, their hands would come out of the coconuts.

"Now, some people will think that it was the rice that was the downfall of these monkeys. No. Others will point to the animal lovers. No. Some will think that it was the monkeys' greed, or perhaps their desire for the rice that made them prisoners. No! I think that it was simply the monkeys' inability to let go. After all, if they were to open up their hands, they would be free now!

"Now there is plenty of time, whenever you are ready to become more deeply relaxed. All

COMMENT

Posture may be associated with altering one's perception.

Therapist merely reinterprets a natural phenomenon to stimulate patients' imagination and creativity.

Once again, therapist alludes to an internal conflict that may be resolved by understanding that the individual is maintaining the struggle. Patients are then offered another way of accomplishing this — making friends with oneself.

The therapist now focuses

INDUCTION

you need to do is merely separate your hands and let them come to rest in your lap (or merely allow yourself to melt deeply in the chair).

"If at any time you need to readjust your posture, to help you go deeper, feel free. After all, you are the one in control!

"You know, it is (was) interesting watching your two hands pressing against each other. If I were to ask you before you went into this trance if you were left-handed or right-handed, you would have indicated that you were one or the other. But as I am (was) absorbed in your hands, I see (saw) your hands staying pretty near the center of your body. One would think that if you were right-handed, your hands would move to the left because of the stronger force. And if you were left-handed, they would move to the right. But they stay (stayed) right in the middle. I find that interesting . . . mmmm.

"Well, it seems there is always something more to learn about ourselves. Perhaps, rather than believing that one hand is stronger or more dominant than the other, one could believe that our hands just complement each other. I wonder that if we have a thought, a feeling, or a belief, we don't also have a thought, a feeling, or a belief that is different and yet equal in force, equal in magnitude. Although it may initially appear to be opposite, it may be there to create a balance. After all, what is the sound of one hand clapping? Now, how do you deal with an equal and different force, feeling, thought? Perhaps you can shake hands with it, that's one way of making a friend! I know that when I write with my right hand, I need my left hand to hold down the paper. Plenty of time — just keep on relaxing very deeply.

"I remember the last time we got together,

COMMENT

on patients' ability to exert control over themselves.

Therapist should assume that patients have learned self-hypnosis.

Therapist asks open ended and rhetorical question so that patients may think about answering it.

Deepening techniques which are essentially created by patients themselves.

Therapist emphasizes patient responsibility. Patients begin to associate countdown with going into a deeper trance.

INDUCTION

and you were able to lower your blood pressure, change your breathing into a comfortable rhythm, create a very slow peaceful beating of your heart, yes. Now, before you began to learn self-hypnosis, if I had asked you to accomplish any of these things, you would have given me a confused and perplexed look. But you have already done it. For even now, as you are sitting comfortably in that chair, you may or may not have realized it already, but the rhythm of your breathing has changed. It has become more comfortable — slower — more   at   peace — and it is a good rhythm. Your whole bodily process is changing to meet your new level of comfort!

"And, yes, you have done all that. As I told you before, I will only ask you to do those things that you are capable of doing. The question is, how much are you capable of controlling in your body.

"And now each time, as you inhale and exhale, you might be surprised to find yourself more and more comfortable, more and more relaxed than you have felt in a long, long time. Almost with each breath, you become more at ease, the tension, the tightness, pain, discomfort can drain from your body. That's right! Good.

"And as you allow yourself to become more aware of how relaxed and comfortable you are, you might begin to remember another time, another place when you were so relaxed — so comfortable (pause). Now only if you wish, you might recall this favorite relaxing place and really feel how good it is to be there, yes — only if you want to do so. Now, it doesn't really matter that I know where it is, and you don't even have to tell me about it later. For what is important to you, you are the one to decide, yes.

"And as you imagine whatever you need to

COMMENT	INDUCTION

COMMENT

INDUCTION

experience in order to relax deeply, I shall count down from ten to one.

"And as you hear the numbers going down you will feel yourself going deeper and deeper and you may also notice that your favorite place will become clearer and more real to you, and when I reach the number one, you will be even more relaxed and pleasantly hypnotized.

Again, therapist synchro-nizes the numbers with patients' exhalations of breath.

"Ten, nine . . . deeper and deeper . . . eight, at your own pace and at your own rate, seven, more and more relaxed . . . six, calm, a full person in every way . . . five, halfway there, you are doing very well, four (soft voice) gently, peaceful, three . . . deeper and deeper . . . twooo, comfortable and . . . one . . . good. You are doing very well!

"Now, as you are sitting there in a relaxed state, feeling very much at ease and at peace with yourself, I would like to explain some-thing to you. I want you to enjoy feeling very comfortable. In fact, if you want to, you can

Patients are encouraged to relax and allow un-conscious learning to transpire.

enjoy yourself so much you can let your unconscious mind listen to me while your con-scious mind can continue to relax, and com-fortably think about that very pleasant place, your favorite peaceful place, because many of the things that I want to assist you in accom-plishing are governed by your unconscious mind. Continue as you are, comfortable, calm, and at the right time you will become aware of how to take care of your concerns, all of those that you need to deal with here.

"Now I am going to discuss your concerns and I believe you are going to enjoy the way I present them to you. I will sketch them in general and I want you to realize that I am going to ask of you only the things that are actually possible for you to do.

Goal setting.

"If I were to ask you what your goals are in coming here, you would know some of them quite well, while I'm sure that there are other

COMMENT	INDUCTION

goals you have that are not as clear. For frequently when we set out to accomplish some goals, we find that we achieve more than we imagine; interesting isn't it — yes. So, only if you would like, why don't you take a few moments to review what you would like to achieve — and will achieve — from now on. Yes (therapist pauses).

Attainment of goals will occur.

"I'm sure that you understand that your unconscious mind has a tremendous capacity for learning, and as you continue to relax more deeply your new learnings automatically become an integral part of your total personality. You will respond to ideas and suggestions that are most helpful in establishing a new point of view, a new orientation, a new way of life. That's something you want, isn't it? Relief and release — yes, deeply relaxed.

More than a headache.

Headaches can be controlled when patients decide to master them.

"Imagine the rest of your life without your usual headache, because from now on you will begin to notice a change in the usual pattern of your headache and you will never have that same headache again. Your headaches will become less frequent and less severe — less frequent and less severe — until they disappear — and they *will* disappear, when *you* decide they will.

Different perspective and new attitude.

"Your attempts in the past to relieve your headaches developed tension, anxiety, and frustration. That is all over, now! Now you have the wonderful opportunity to associate relaxation of body and mind with the relief of headaches. You will find yourself having a more comfortable attitude, more confidence in handling your ability to control sensations in your head.

More than a headache; patients imagine life without constant pain.

"After all, I am sure that you have the ability to imagine yourself without your usual headache, how your life would be different, how it would feel to be relieved — Mmmm. For a long time it may have felt, it may even still feel, that your headache is a constant com-

COMMENT	INDUCTION

INDUCTION

panion. Now if I were to ask you if your headache is part of yourself like your heart, back or even your head, you would respond that, of course, you can live without this ache but you need your heart, your back, your head. After all, you are more than just a headache, much more. So, you could still be yourself without having this pain — relaxing very deeply, good.

Can patients allow headache to leave?

"And as I talk to you, you will absorb what I say deeply into yourself. As you are learning how to relax deeply and utilize the resources that are deep within you, you are developing more confidence in yourself — realizing that you are capable of so much — more than you thought yourself capable of. After all, you are sitting in the chair exceedingly comfortably, very much at ease and in comfort. And you enjoy your ability to attain this peaceful and calm awareness — just by allowing yourself to become aware of the vast reservoir that is deep within you. For you have already achieved so much, haven't you? And how did you do it? Perhaps by trusting yourself — for all I am doing is talking — and you have allowed yourself to experience how wonderful you feel when you are relaxed, yes.

Ego strengthening suggestions building on patients' accomplishments of:

self-hypnosis,

self-trust,

"And as you continue to feel comfortable and enjoy how wonderful it feels to be here, experience your favorite relaxing place. You may tell yourself that you can return anytime you wish — that's right, simply by taking a few moments to relax yourself and letting your imagination, your memories, carry you here. Each time you come to visit, you will find it more peaceful, even more serene than you remember it to be, and more comfortable as new horizons are opened for you to experience.

self-control,

and self-realization.

Therapist reassures patients that they will achieve their goals.

"It is so easy — so accessible — so available to you even when you are no longer with me. For my voice will be with you — it will be the voice of a friend — it will be the voice of a gentle breeze — it will be the voice of the

COMMENT	INDUCTION

rain, the voice of the wind and yes, the voice of the sun!

"And just to show you that you can achieve what you set out to do, and that you are able to use hypnosis to help you, in a few moments, I will say the word "now." When I say this word, you will begin to count to yourself from one to ten. As the numbers increase, you will feel yourself becoming more and more alert. And when you say the number "ten," you will open your eyes, and come out of the trance feeling alert, refreshed and also very comfortably relaxed. And tonight when you go to sleep, you will really be able to enjoy the comfort of your bed, you will have a very deep and restful sleep, like one you had a long . . . long . . . time ago. And you will awaken in the morning feeling calm and secure, rested, comfortable and confident. Yes, confident in your ability to easily go into and come out of a trance, and to comfortably carry out this treatment. Good, easier and easier.

"Now, it is up to you, at your own pace and at your own rate. Good."

Familiar pattern of hypnotic state coming to an end so patients can awaken themselves at their own pace.

THIRD SESSION

THIRD SESSION

COMMENT

Patients should be informed about any forthcoming changes in procedure, and that the fourth session will be the last treatment session. (This is, of course, subject to change.)

Preview — As in the previous session, the format will be as follows:

- Review of reactions to last treatment session (refer to second paragraph of Session Two for more detail of what to explore with patients).
- "How are you today?" and "Have there been any changes in headaches, sleep patterns, medication intake, daily activities," etc.
- Obtain reactions to last induction, reinforce any positive reactions, remember to discard what patient dislikes.
- Ask if patients have practiced at all, etc., if applicable.

In this session, the therapist should convey a message of reassurance that patients will do very well. After all, this time they will be essentially utilizing their own approaches to relax and hypnotize themselves. The therapist's behavior and language should convey to patients that hypnosis is now accessible to them.

After patient feedback and/or questions, the following procedure is initiated:

COMMENT

Pre induction.

All hypnosis is self-hypnosis. Therapist has guided patients in exploring and realizing their own potentials.

INDUCTION

"That's right, you can get as comfortable as you wish in that chair. Before you develop a very pleasant hypnotic state, I'm going to discuss what will happen today. You have already demonstrated your ability to deeply relax and to respond to suggestions very well.

"Now, we will go one step further. You will go into a trance without guidance from me. For now, you have a skill that has become part of you, that you can rely on, whether it is in relaxing comfortably and deeply, in graciously handling headaches, alleviating excess tension, pain, discomfort or for whatever you

COMMENT	INDUCTION

COMMENT

Can make use of hypnosis in many ways.

Preparing patients for forthcoming glove anesthesia.

By this point, patients know how to hypnotize themselves.

Brief summary of different inductions used:

1. One arm lever.

2. Both hands clasped together.

3. Deep breathing.

4. Countdown.

Individuals may have their preferences for going into a trance.

INDUCTION

choose to apply it.

"I know someone who learned hypnosis for controlling his fear of speaking in front of groups. Well, he did very well at that, but what is also interesting is that he once got a sharp metal splinter in the palm of his hand. Ouch! Whew, that's a sensitive spot. Well, he went into a deep trance, numbed his whole hand so he wouldn't experience the pain, and then his wife proceeded to remove the splinter. His wife was amazed and couldn't believe it, and he was relieved of the splinter.

"So who knows the limits of what you learn here. I'm sure that you have heard of people who have lost weight, stopped smoking, alleviated unnecessary anxiety, and relieved pain with hypnosis. The tools are now with you, the house you build is up to you.

"Now, in a little while, whenever you are ready to enter a deep trance, just close your eyes and go into a very comfortable and pleasant hypnotic state. Now, I have shown you a number of ways of doing this. The first time we got together, you utilized the one arm lever approach, combined with your staring at your arm. The second time, you used both of your hands clasped tightly together and then you imagined yourself in your favorite relaxing place.

"Another way is to recognize that your breathing is slowing down as you go into a trance. A variation of this approach is to combine the counting down from ten to one with your exhalation of breath. So every time you breathe out, you will count down, and on the tenth breath, you will be comfortably and deeply relaxed.

"You may use any of these techniques, or perhaps you have one of your own that you enjoy and is equally effective in developing a nice trance state. It is entirely up to you what you choose to use. You know what works best for you.

"Any questions before you go into a trance?"

COMMENT

Once again, it is important to remember to encourage a positive response set for patients. Use a tone, mood, and attitude that convey a supportive reassuring message that patients will succeed. Keep on "being with the patients." Remember to use their behavior, attitudes, feelings, even skepticism as either the starting point or the result of being good subjects.

Any feedback from patients about what they liked and disliked in the previous induction; i.e., words, scenes, voice quality, etc., will be useful additions to this induction. Being aware of patients' present emotional state is also helpful. Modifying your style to reflect patients' unique characteristics can only add more credibility to your induction.

COMMENT

Induction. Familiar pattern associated with going into trance.

Patients are encouraged to focus on the important messages communicated, through an indirect reference to the unconscious learning that will transpire.

Therapist explains ideo-motor signaling and uses this method as a double bind for demonstrating to patients that they will be in a self-induced hypnotic trance.

INDUCTION

"Now, if anyone comes to the door, or if the phone rings, just leave it to me. I know that you can hear any sounds that you wish (slowly mention sounds presently in environment), but the only important thing for you right now is the sound of my voice and the meaning of what I have to say to you; so you really don't need to give any attention to anything else unless you have a particular interest in (refer to sounds already mentioned).

"One other thing before you begin: I won't speak until you signal to me that you are in a deep hypnotic trance. Instead of telling me when you have achieved this, just move one of your fingers. Which finger would you prefer to use? (Wait until patient demonstrates and then say) O.K.; when I see that finger move, I will know that you are comfortably, pleasantly relaxed and deeply hypnotized. At that time, I will begin to speak, and the sound

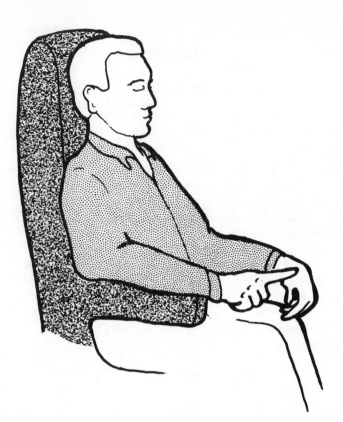

Patient signals with one finger that he has reached a deep trance state.

COMMENT	INDUCTION
	of my voice will help you to feel even more comfortable. O.K.? (Wait until patient indicates understanding either by a nod of the head or verbal assurance.) I will continue to speak to you, and I will help you by offering suggestions that will be of help to you. All you will need to do is to relax deeply.
Therapist reassures that there is plenty of time. . . .	"Now, there is plenty of time, plenty of time — you will do very well. Whenever you are ready to deeply relax and be pleasantly hypnotized, you may begin. It is now up to you." (Therapist stares straight ahead, while patient initiates the induction. The manner and mood of the therapist should convey the

COMMENT	INDUCTION

COMMENT

*Patients have acknowl-
edged being in a trance.*

Deepening technique.

*Can patients allow them-
selves to be aware of how
relaxed they feel?*

*Therapist challenges
patients to use their
imagination to prove
to themselves that they
are hypnotized.*

INDUCTION

belief that the patient will be able to accomplish it.)

(Long pause — patient moves a finger.)

"O.K. you can rest your finger and enjoy
the comfort of relaxing very deeply, and being
pleasantly hypnotized.

"First of all, I want you to enjoy feeling very
comfortable." At this point refer to whatever
activity the patient is exhibiting and note how
this indicates being deeply relaxed; i.e.,
"Good, as you swallow, smile, breathe easier,
etc. you feel a deep sense of relaxation and
comfort flowing throughout your body. This
delightful feeling of relaxation is spreading
through the muscles of your face, your brow,
your neck, your shoulders, and downward
through your chest, your back melting like
butter into the chair. Allowing the chair to
hold you, feel the peaceful comfort down
through your stomach, thighs, legs, toes. You
are becoming more and more deeply, yes
deeply, relaxed. If at any time you need to
adjust your posture, feel free, because I would
like you to enjoy feeling very comfortable.
Can you allow yourself to be aware of how
deeply relaxed you are? Yes. And now you
can enjoy the comfort (pause) of going even
deeper into the trance.

"In a while, I am going to ask you to imagine that a bright, intense beam of light is
shining directly into your eyes. Perhaps you
will tell yourself it is glaring sunlight shining
into your eyes; maybe you will imagine someone holding a bright flashlight in front of your
eyes. Whatever you imagine, you will sense it
as a glaring, bright light shining directly in
your eyes. It is, of course, very difficult to
open your eyes as you imagine this.

"I am going to ask you to try and open your
eyes as you imagine this. Yes, to try, to try to
open your eyes, but you won't be able to,
because the harder you try, the more they

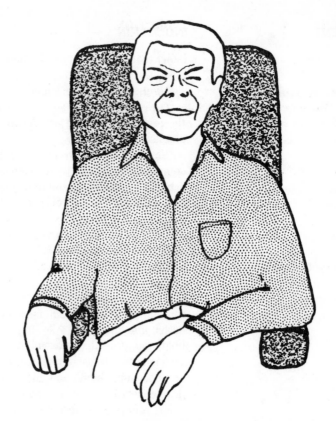

Patient imagines glaring light shining in his eyes.

COMMENT

INDUCTION

Patients imagine light; now try to open their eyes.

will want to stay closed.

"So, (patient's name), now imagine and tell yourself that a bright ray of glaring light is shining in your eyes, glaring bright light directly in your eyes — and try, yes, try to open them, but you won't be able to because the harder you try, the more they want to stay closed. Try, try in the glaring light." (Choose whatever response is applicable. If patient responds by struggling to open eyes, but they remain closed, use sections 1 and 2. If the patient responds by opening eyes easily, use section 2 only.)

1. After about ten seconds of the patient's eyes being closed, say "O.K., relax. You did

COMMENT	INDUCTION

COMMENT

Power of the mind.

Inner resources.

Patients' eyes open while in trance.

Therapist uses patient behavior as a basis for deepening techniques. Circumvent conscious resistance with unconscious learning.

Patients' own way of experiencing hypnosis.

Eyes closed.

Patients can allow themselves comfort, ease and realization of potentials to help themselves.

Self healing.

INDUCTION

fine. Now, relax deeply. The light is gone, the sun went behind a cloud. Relax. You have demonstrated by your ability to do that, that by the power of your mind, you are able to exert control over your body. Good! You have within you the ability to relax, to imagine, to utilize your own inner resources to control your bodily processes. Yes, just to show you that you can open your eyes and remain in a deep trance, open your eyes now, the intense light is gone."

2. When the patient's eyes are open, say "That's fine. Now just look about the room and pick some small spot to look at steadily as you continue to relax deeply with your eyes open. Look at any spot. Yes, just keep looking at that spot. That's right, good. You really don't even need to pay attention to me. You can enjoy this so much that you can allow your unconscious mind to listen to me while your conscious mind can continue to relax deeply, deeply. For after all, your unconscious mind will hear me. And while you have been sitting there, you have been letting your body breathe itself, using its own natural rhythm — slowly — easily — and deeply. This is your own way of acknowledging the experience of relaxation and comfort. Now you may imagine or project on that spot, your favorite relaxing place, as you close your eyes, now!

"You can now enjoy the quiet comfort of going ever deeper into a trance. I want you to enjoy being very comfortable, and you can even allow yourself to become aware of the ease, the comforts, the resources, and even the potentials within yourself. Then, perhaps you will have the experience of sensing as you relax the experience of healing, restoring, nourishing yourself.

"From now on, you have as your resource the ability to release tension, release the tight-

COMMENT	INDUCTION

Self hypnosis.   ness, and enjoy this very pleasant state of relaxation by just opening up your hands (or by raising and then lowering your hand)."

COMMENT

The rationale for this particular procedure is for patients to demonstrate to themselves their ability to elicit a self-hypnotic trance. Furthermore, including a challenge (eye closure) after they have already acknowledged that they are in a deep trance (by ideomotor signaling) provides a basis for the subsequent glove anesthesia. At this point, patients are essentially convinced that they can attain self-hypnosis.

The reader will note that there are two options for the therapist to choose in response to patients' reactions to the suggestion of eye closure. This is to provide patients with the opportunity of experiencing hypnosis in a manner congruent with their particular needs. If patients need to open their eyes, or keep them closed, the therapist can continue, as he/she has done throughout the entire treatment procedure, reaffirming that patients are responsible for their own behavior.

At this point in the treatment procedure, a glove anesthesia technique is introduced to patients, while they are in a trance. The patients are told to continue relaxing, but also to attend and follow the therapist's instructions.

There are many ways of utilizing and demonstrating glove anesthesia to patients. The critical premise for this approach is that patients experience a numbness in one of their hands and then transfer this feeling to the affected part of their bodies. In this example, individuals would bring their hands to their heads and then either massage or stroke the painful area. Having patients focus their attention on one of their hands and then the therapist's suggesting that a certain feeling will be experienced such as numbness, tingling, or throbbing, will generally result in patient confirmation of this phenomenon.

This is really quite simple to achieve. The reader, for instance, could stop reading and begin focusing attention on one hand; within a short period of time one will become aware of sensations in that area. It is basically focusing one's attention and then labeling that experience. The reason we utilize this approach in the treatment is that patients are given the opportunity to do something about their pain rather than experiencing helplessness. Patients may use this

COMMENT

as a distraction technique, or perhaps in some way they may define, to alleviate their discomfort. Once again, we are emphasizing patient responsibility for their perception of pain.

COMMENT	INDUCTION

Glove anesthesia technique.

"Now, as you continue to relax deeply and enjoy the comfort of this very pleasant and deep hypnotic state, I would like to explain something to you. You remember at the beginning of today's session I mentioned a person who learned hypnosis for controlling his fear of speaking in front of groups, and he did very well at that. He was also able to use hypnosis to help numb his hand when he hurt it so he wouldn't experience the pain as his wife removed a splinter.

"Now, I am going to show you a way that you can use a similar approach to help you in controlling your pain and discomfort. With your eyes remaining closed, and while remaining deeply hypnotized and pleasantly relaxed, I would like for you to imagine a small table being placed in front of you on which there are some items. Good. I will describe three possible items on the small table; there may be more or less — that depends on you.

Imagery that essentially focuses on a textural perception.
Imagery that essentially focuses on a visual perception.
Imagery that essentially focuses on olfactory perception.

"The first object is a beautiful, soft, velvet glove with a smooth silk lining.

"The second object is a pail — a new, brightly colored pail, filled with a sparkling, blue liquid.

"The third object is a large jar of hand cream, and the jar is open, revealing a most pleasant and aromatic perfume, mmmm.

Self control and then self mastery.

"Now, I don't know what you are able to imagine, or which of these items seems most interesting to you, but if you proceed as if they are real, you may be surprised to discover that the relief you will experience will

-39-

COMMENT	INDUCTION

COMMENT

The therapist should repeat the name of the object that patients choose, so he/she is able to align suggestions with the specific choice.

The following instructions can be adapted to any one of the objects or to what-ever patients may imagine. The key is focusing patients' attention on their ability to control their perception of the sensations.

Patients are aware of feelings and therapist uses their perception to suggest various phenomena.

INDUCTION

also be real.

"You see, each one of these objects contains an extremely potent anesthesia, that alleviates pain by numbing an area of your body. I'm sure that in your lifetime you have felt a numbness, perhaps a tingling — maybe when you went to the dentist and were given novocaine so you wouldn't feel the pain — a feeling of numbness. That's right.

"While remaining pleasantly relaxed, now, and deeply hypnotized, I want you to pick up one of these objects off the small table in front of you. It doesn't matter which one you choose; that is entirely up to you. However, I am interested in your choice, so could you please tell what it is, while remaining relaxed and hypnotized.

"Now that you have chosen (the object chosen), place your hand inside of it, which-ever hand you prefer." Wait until patient makes hand gesture and then say, "That's right, you are doing very well. As you place your left (or right) hand in (the object chosen, i.e., silk glove, aromatic cream, pail of spar-kling blue liquid) feel your fingertips tingle as the anesthetic is quickly absorbed. Slowly place your hand in more comfortably, more securely. Allow yourself to experience the numbness up to your knuckles, across your palm and the back of your hand. That's right, really allow yourself to experience this, for as you proceed through these actions, you will become aware that the relief you experience will also be real.

"Now, I don't know exactly what you are experiencing in your hand. You are the one who is aware of sensations like numbness, tingling, gentleness. As the potent anesthetic seeps even deeper, the skin on your hand will feel even more constricted, much more numb. That's right. Can you sense the movement of the remaining feelings in your hand as they

-40-

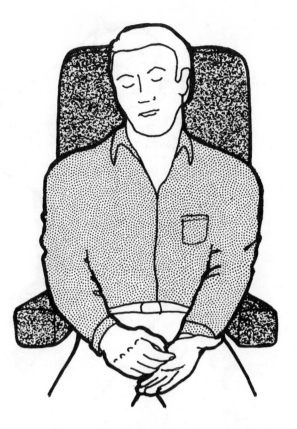

Patient places his hand into "anesthetic."

COMMENT

INDUCTION

Double bind of placing hand on head and then exchanging tension for comfort.

glide out of your fingertips into (the object chosen)? Continue to experience this and in a while I will ask you to gently place your left (or right) hand on your head. This will give you the opportunity to transfer the feelings of numbness in your hand directly to your head, where you usually experience a headache, and in exchange, any tension, tightness, pain or discomfort will flow from your head into your hand. Good.

"You can now begin to gently touch, massage or stroke your head, and allow the sensations to transfer from your hand to your head." When patient begins to do this, you

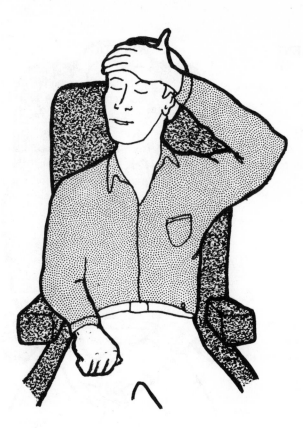

Patient transfers sensations of numbness from hand to head.

COMMENT

Question of whether patients can allow themselves to become aware of other feelings they can experience.

INDUCTION

say, "Yes, that's right, allow all the deep feelings of numbness to flow from your hand into your head. The same feelings are now gently seeping into your head. Can you allow yourself to experience that once painful area feeling better and more comfortable? I wonder if you are aware of the differences in sensations that have already occurred. Slowly and effortlessly stroke your hand around your head. As you allow the combination of numbness and relaxation to penetrate all over, experience how good this feels.

"You can repeat the transfer process as many times as you want to, and each time you will feel an even greater amount of comfort

COMMENT	INDUCTION

COMMENT

INDUCTION

and relief than you did before. And each time you repeat it, you will find it easier and easier."

Therapist emphasizes natural feelings returning to patients' hands.

Therapist pauses. "Whenever you are ready to conclude this particular procedure, remove your hand from your head and simply shake your hand briskly for a few seconds and all the natural feelings will return to it. You will remain pleasantly relaxed and deeply hypnotized." When patient has done as instructed, you say, "Good. After doing this you may be surprised to notice that you continue not only to feel relaxed and comfortable, but confident in your ability to achieve the goals you have set for yourself.

Ego strengthening techniques building on patients' accomplishments of:

"As you allow yourself to relax, you will fully absorb what I am saying. You will be able to remember what is important for you to remember.

self relaxation,

"As you learn how to relax deeply and utilize the resources within you, you are developing more confidence in your abilities and potentials, and realizing that you are capable of so much more than you thought yourself capable of. After all, you are sitting comfortably in the chair, very much at ease.

self hypnosis,

And you enjoy your ability to attain this peaceful and calm state of awareness. As you continue to remember and use what you find helpful here, you will discover that it becomes

self mastery,

easier and easier, and the relief you achieve will last longer and longer. As you become more confident in yourself you will no longer fear your headache, because you will no longer allow it to control your way of life. You

self trust,

have achieved so much already, just by allowing yourself to become aware of the vast resources that are deep within you. You have sensed within yourself a wholeness, a feeling

self realization,

of discovering something special, meaningful, and fulfilling within yourself.

self control,

"While you are relaxing and enjoying how

COMMENT	INDUCTION

wonderful it feels to be comfortable, peaceful, and at ease, tell yourself that you can return any time you wish simply by taking a few moments to relax yourself and letting your imagination — your memories — carry you there. Each time you come to visit you will find it more peaceful, more serene, more natural and more invigorating than you

and increased learning.

remembered it to be, as new horizons are opened for you to experience.

Remember a positive experience anytime.

"It is so easy, so accessible, so available to you even when you are no longer with me. You will remember my voice and what I have told you. It will be the voice of a friend — the voice of a gentle breeze. It will be the voice of the wind — the rain — and yes, the voice of the sun.

Therapist reassurance and then familiar pattern of trance coming to an end when patients are ready to terminate it.

"And just to show you that you can achieve what you set out to, and that you are able to use hypnosis to help you, in a few moments I will say the word "now." When I say this word, you can begin to count to yourself from one to ten. As the numbers increase, you will feel yourself becoming more and more alert. When you say the number "ten," you can open your eyes, and come out of the trance feeling alert, refreshed and comfortably re-

Once again, therapist refers to a good night's sleep, and patients' waking with a renewed sense of confidence in themselves.

laxed. Tonight when you go to sleep, you will really be able to enjoy the comfort of your bed, and have a deep and restful sleep, like one you had a long time ago. And you will awaken in the morning feeling calm and secure, rested, comfortable, and confident. Yes, confident in your ability to easily go into and come out of a trance, and to comfortably carry out your treatment.

"Now! It is up to you, at your own pace and at your own rate. Good."

FOURTH SESSION